YOUR KNOWLEDGE HAS VALUE

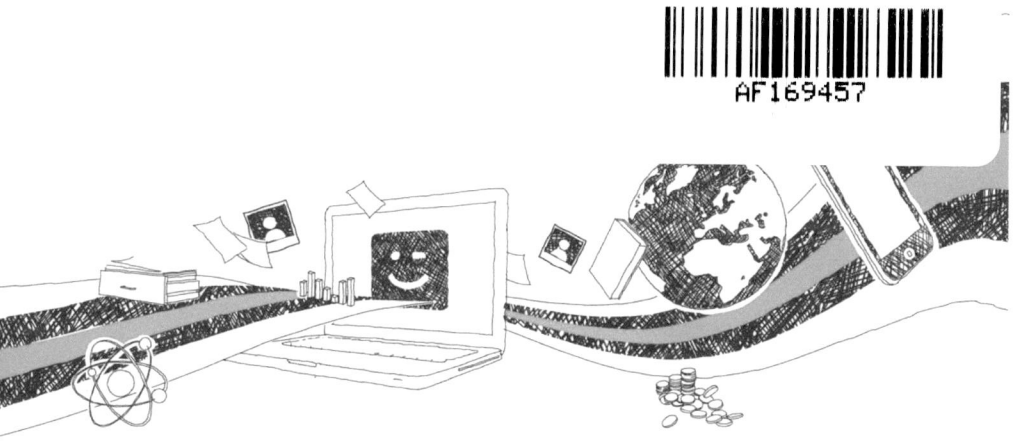

- We will publish your bachelor's and master's thesis, essays and papers

- Your own eBook and book - sold worldwide in all relevant shops

- Earn money with each sale

Upload your text at www.GRIN.com
and publish for free

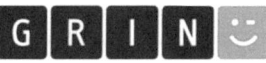

Bibliographic information published by the German National Library:

The German National Library lists this publication in the National Bibliography; detailed bibliographic data are available on the Internet at http://dnb.dnb.de .

This book is copyright material and must not be copied, reproduced, transferred, distributed, leased, licensed or publicly performed or used in any way except as specifically permitted in writing by the publishers, as allowed under the terms and conditions under which it was purchased or as strictly permitted by applicable copyright law. Any unauthorized distribution or use of this text may be a direct infringement of the author s and publisher s rights and those responsible may be liable in law accordingly.

Imprint:

Copyright © 2016 GRIN Verlag, Open Publishing GmbH
Print and binding: Books on Demand GmbH, Norderstedt Germany
ISBN: 9783668363045

This book at GRIN:

http://www.grin.com/en/e-book/346669/donor-conditions-in-hiv-aids-programs-funding-lessons-for-the-poor-recipient

Kibs Boaz Muhanguzi

Donor Conditions in HIV/AIDS Programs' funding. Lessons for the Poor Recipient Countries

GRIN Publishing

GRIN - Your knowledge has value

Since its foundation in 1998, GRIN has specialized in publishing academic texts by students, college teachers and other academics as e-book and printed book. The website www.grin.com is an ideal platform for presenting term papers, final papers, scientific essays, dissertations and specialist books.

Visit us on the internet:

http://www.grin.com/

http://www.facebook.com/grincom

http://www.twitter.com/grin_com

Donor Conditions in HIV/AIDS Program's funding: Lessons for the Poor Recipient Countries

Content

Abstract 1
Introduction 1
Study Purpose 4
Related Literature 5
Key donors in HIV/AIDS programs 5
Key Donor Requirements 6
References 11

Donor Conditions in HIV/AIDS Programs' funding: Lessons for the Poor Recipient Countries

By
Kibs Boaz Muhanguzi[1]

Abstract
Management of HIV/AIDS scourge worldwide attracts financial resources from different donor agencies often with conditions and specific requirements attached. Despite of huge flow of HIV/AIDS funds into poor countries, AIDS related problems remain a menace. Stringent fund conditions and requirements are perceived to impede the struggle against the pandemic. This paper investigates lessons recipient organizations need to learn from donor conditions, if the struggle against HIV/AIDS is to be fully tenable. Guided by existing literature, the study uses a mixed paradigm approach (quantitative and qualitative) with a cross sectional data from both donor and implementing agencies. The study finds an average 29.9% level of non compliance to the 9 investigated donor conditions. Given the implied effects of non compliance to donor conditions and supported with literature review, the study points to two categorical lessons: first, need to invest more on capacity building-particularly, HR training-so as to reduce overreliance on foreign manpower; and second, the need to ensure coordinated programming of funds for harmonious solicitation and funding of HIV/AIDS project activities.

Key words: donor funding, donor conditions, HIV/AIDS programs, recipient countries

Introduction
Donor funding often goes with strings attached. For example, some bilateral donors offer grants to specific organizations with which they have relations. Most multilateral donors channel their

---

[1] Kibs Muhanguzi is currently a Lecturer in the Department of Economics and Statistics, Kampala International University

funds through specific country's line Ministry. Other donations like those by the GHIs are part of the country's central budget. Some grants are conditioned solely to specific activities/programs. Some donors require recipient countries/organization to present technical papers (proposal, budget, M&E reports …) before receiving the first or further funding. When such conditions are not met, funds are withheld. In relation to multifaceted HIV/AIDS programs, this study aims at investigating the level of compliance by recipient countries/organizations and how this influences the struggle to eliminate the pandemic disease. It is from this that lessons are drawn to further the struggle in the fight against the disease.

Since 2000, the global AIDS debate has been dominated by two major issues: first, the rising prevalence levels in some regions (Southern Africa, China, India and the Russian Federation) and second, the claims of the Ugandan miracle-possible causes and lessons for others. Since early 1980's, a number of multi donor agencies have come up to join hands in the fight against HIV/AIDS pandemic in Africa (including musicians).[2] These agencies give conditions on which HIV/AIDS funds are to be accessed. Each donor specializes on a particular activity: some specialize in funding HIV/AIDS prevention through donating condoms; others fund health care, treatment, while others fund campaigns to sensitize the public. The HIV/AIDS funding has been so important internationally, though it has rarely been subjected to careful scrutiny, especially in matters related to aid conditions.

As HIV/AIDS epidemic matured, expenditure requirements were spreading to include not only prevention and social mobilization, but care and support (Whelan, 2001). This mandated the role of international partnerships against the disease and international financial commitments were doubled in Africa in the year 2000. Barnet et al. (2001) observes that in many developing countries, NGOs have taken a lead in responding to HIV/AIDS crisis. As international funding has increased, donors and government officials are looking for effective ways to distribute new funding to maximize impact. Contracting was found to be one of the more effective ways of introducing performance-based systems into HIV/AIDS program. However, challenges include the need for resources to plan and implement a contracting program, political resistance and lack of capacity among NGOs.

There are three main categorical sources of HIV/AIDS funding: first is the 'the Global Health Initiatives GHIs' with key organizations like; The Global Fund for Aids, Tuberculosis and Malaria ATM; USAID's President's Emergency Plan for AIDS Relief PEPFAR; and the World Bank's Multi-country AIDS Program (MAP). Second is 'multilateral agencies' like the World Health Organization (WHO), the United Nations Children's Fund (UNICEF), the Joint United Nations Program on HIV/AIDS (UNAIDS) and the World Bank. And third is 'bilateral agencies' like Japan International Cooperation Agency, the Norwegian Agency for Development (NORAD), and the United States Agency for International Development (USAID), and the United Kingdom's Department for International Development (DFID), the Swedish International Development Cooperation Agency (SIDA) and the Danish International Development Agency (DANIDA). Some Health Development Partners indirectly fund HIV/AIDS through their direct

---

[2] Also see appendix 3-a song by Philly Lutaaya

support to the general budget like the Belgian Technical Cooperation (BTC), the Netherlands, and the German Technical Agency for Development (GTZ).

Following Nabyonga et al (2009) article, the following issues were raised about aid funds: Predictability: Donors provide project budget figures at the beginning of the budget cycle and efforts are made as much as possible to discuss priorities to be funded between the donors and the Ministry of Health. Channeling of donor funds: We note that funds are channeled through both public and private entities. Although private entities play a role in service delivery, they must be regulated and supervised to ensure that they are contributing to sector objectives. Alignment to priorities: Donor funds must be properly aligned to HIV/AIDS program priorities to ensure maximum benefits. Fiscal sustainability: As developing countries continue to receive donor aid for health, they should also ensure mobilization of domestic resources.

Tracking the flow of funding for HIV/AIDS programs in poor countries proves challenging for several reasons: none of the donors publicly discloses all of the funding data that would be required to truly trace monies from source to ultimate use; HIV/AIDS monies are used in a broad range of sectors, from health to education to transportation and mining, complicating the task of sorting out both amounts and uses; the funding flows through a diverse set of channels – some within the public accounting system in-country and some outside of it – making it hard to account for all funds; and finally, the in-country researchers encounter difficulties in gaining access to and information from some government and donor officials. Nevertheless, research into donor conditions, level of compliance to these conditions, and the implied effect on HIV/AIDS program effectiveness is partly made possible using survey of related literature as this paper delves into. For example, figure 1.1 shows a 4-year proportion of donor funding in HIV/AIDS programs in Uganda.

In Uganda, various donors contribute huge resources directly to the HIV/AIDS programs. These include USAID, DFID, DANIDA, CIDA, SIDA and IBRD. Most NGOs get their share of funding directly from donors and then do accountability for the funds to the respective donors. Conditions for access and accountability are made known to the grantee before release of funds. This is the reason HIV/AIDS programs tap into different sources of funds to implement their activities (Riddell, 2002).

Figure 1.1 Major donors in HIV/AIDS project activities in Uganda (2003/04 -2006/07)

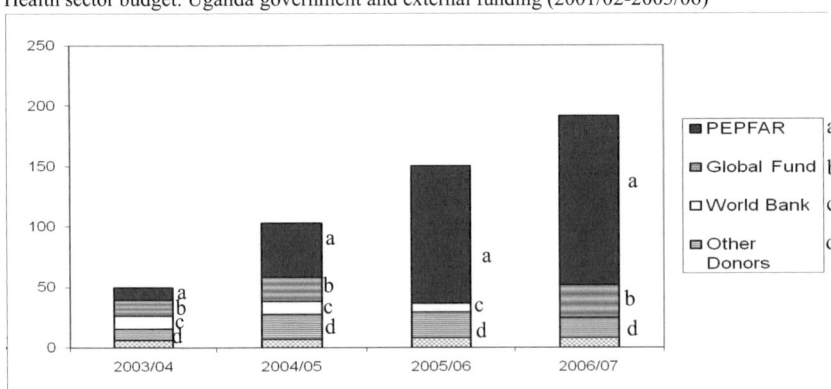

Health sector budget: Uganda government and external funding (2001/02-2005/06)

Source: Lake, sector-based assessment of HIV/AIDS spending in Uganda, 2006

Donor funding demands accountability (Harshmat, 2004) which lies at the core of NGOs function because of the nature of their relations with diverse stakeholders. The government provides legal cover while donors provide finance to NGOs to work with communities. Hence, NGOs are faced with the diverse requirements of accountability in trends of reporting financial situation and progress to each stakeholder, thereby making accountability mechanisms more complex. Multi-donor funded programs find it costly to hire auditors to express an opinion on different sets of fund accountability statements. For example, TASO Uganda must have a minimum of 4 audited statements: USAID, EU, CDC and general purpose accounts for general assembly. This arrangement takes a lot of time in preparation attending to auditors and has increased costs. TASO has tried to minimize on time taken by appointing one audit firm to carry out external audit of all fund accountability statements, but some donor agencies like EU prefer to hire their own auditors as a condition for funding. According to TASO (1994) memorandum and articles of association (Article 8 section 7), BOT members are only empowered to recommend auditors to the general assembly for appointment (TASO, 2001)

Though the ultimate goal of recipient countries and donors is to efficiently and effectively utilize the available resources for prevention and reduction of the spread of HIV/AIDS, some donor requirements inhibit this noble purpose (Mosisilli, 2001). In Uganda, HIV/AIDS implementing agencies deal in a variety of activities for example; prevention, treatment, palliative care, sensitization, and research.

It is believed that the conditions and requirements set by the donors for implementing agencies before they access funds, often make it so hard for implementing agencies to make good use of these funds save so much exorbitant expenses they make on hiring external technicians: auditors, accountants, monitoring and evaluation officers, procurement and contracting officers. Often times, the donors dictate who to run what, by sending their own personnel experts who are paid a very big fraction of the funds donated.

Study Purpose
The purpose of this study is to identify lessons recipient countries should learn from the effect of donor conditions on HIV/AIDS funding towards program implementation.

Related literature
For donor aid to be effective several prerequisites must be in place, including fiscal sustainability of the wider reform program, sustainability of aided development projects, predictability, fungibility, and absorptive capacity (Nabyonga etal, 2009). Other preconditions that must be in place include local ownership of development strategies and effective stewardship of governments, improved donor coordination, stronger partnerships, results-based approach, capacity building, and engaging civil society. Equally important is the commitment from donors to align to government plans and use government structures. Although NGOs and CSOs are important providers of health care and significant proportions of donor funds are channeled through them, effective regulatory mechanisms must be in place to ensure that these contribute towards agreed health sector strategies. There is need for partnerships between donors and the NGOs/CBOs and government so as to ensure: sustainability, capacity building and training within the organization, including training of staff and volunteers; training in monitoring and evaluation skills; office space and infrastructure (including telephone lines) from which to manage growing operations; building linkages between organizations.

Key donors in HIV/AIDS programs
1. The US Presidential Emergence Program For Aids Response PEPFAR[3]

PEPFAR Funding is largely allocated based on requirements set by the U.S. Congress for the treatment, prevention, and care of patients as well as orphans and vulnerable children. The recipient organizations are chosen largely by their ability to meet targets, and have few capacity constraints. They fund mainly internationally non-governmental entities based in the US. Some money is transferred to recipient governments, and funding is managed and overseen by U.S. government personnel. The annual process for preparing the country operational plan is very time-consuming, requiring the full attention of PEPFAR staff as well as substantial time from the staff in the recipient organizations.

2. The Global Fund Aids Tuberculosis and Malaria ATM

Recognized stakeholders in recipient countries determine which programs get Global Fund money. The money is usually disbursed to the national government. It is spent according to country-designed procedures and by country-selected recipients. Common bottlenecks of this fund emanate primarily from lack of capacity to manage funds by the recipient organizations.

3. The World Bank MAP

MAP funding uniquely focuses on strengthening the national AIDS response by allocating its money to particular types of recipients, such as National AIDS Councils; it also places priority on capacity building and institutional strengthening rather than particular programmatic areas, such as prevention, treatment, or care. All MAP funding is disbursed first to the national government, but money is spent according to MAP-specific procedures aimed at ensuring the proper use of funds. MAP funding encounters significant bottlenecks moving through the

---

[3] Following the funding for HIV/AIDS: A comparative analysis the of funding practices of PEPFAR, the Global fund and World Bank's MAP in Uganda, Zambia and Mozambique, October 10, 2007 by Oomman Nandini, BernStein Micheal, Rosenzweing Steven.

government system because of a combination of extensive procedural and reporting requirements, overburdened government staff, and bureaucratic entanglement.

4. World Health Organization (WHO):

The WHO global program on AIDS (GPA) ceased operations on 31 December 1995. WHO/GPA was the major recipient of multi-lateral and multi-bilateral funding for HIV/AIDS between 1987 and 1995. WHO's HIV/AIDS priorities include the prevention, detection and treatment of STDs; the prevention of sexual transmission of HIV; the transmission of HIV through blood; the reduction of transmission associated with substance abuse; the prevention of prenatal transmission of HIV; the care and support of persons or groups affected by HIV/AIDS/TB and STDs based on the strengthening of health care systems; and the promotion of adequate and appropriate social responses to HIV/AIDS.

5. UNESCO–United Nations Educational, Scientific and Cultural Organizations

Although not a funding agency, UNESCO contributes to the work in the area of HIV/AIDS by virtue of the scope of its fields of competence and approaches. UNESCO has also funded activities focused on preventive education and basic science and research in the area of HIV/AIDS in the areas of gender, communication and ethics and human rights.

Basis for donor conditions are; first, HIV prevalence; people in charge of disbursement of money can be drawn to those areas that have the highest prevalence of people infected with HIV. Whilst these areas certainly have the greatest need, this does not mean that other areas in which HIV prevalence is lower do not have the same needs. It can be as valuable to work in areas where the impact of HIV is not as evident as elsewhere. Second, geography: Some donors tend to favor certain geographical areas. This may be because these areas have a higher media-coverage than others, because these areas are safer than others for staff to visit, or it may simply be because these areas have better amenities for staff that might prefer to travel in comfort. Whatever the reason, there are geographical inequalities in spending, with some regions having sufficient funds and others having almost none. Third, perceptions of good governance: Acute need can be overlooked when a political situation is off-putting for donors. Civil war, a collapsed or corrupt government and widespread violence can lead to decreased assistance. For example, UNITAID, the World Bank and PEPFAR plan to withdraw from the war ravaged state of the Democratic Republic of Congo in 2011. This is despite increased need for antiretroviral treatment (only 10 % of people needing treatment in the DRC receive it - far less than in other parts of sub-Saharan Africa). Fifth, type of HIV work: Different types of HIV work attract different levels of funding. Sometimes, funding will be made available for AIDS treatment, for example, but not for staff training. Often, donors are reluctant to give significant assistance to stigmatized and marginalized groups such as sex workers and injecting drug users, even if these are the people most affected by HIV (Guthrie & Hickey, 2004).

Key Donor Requirements

1. Contracting and awarding of grants

Barnet et.al (2001) shows that "at national level, donors and funding units are predominantly concerned with identifying and funding NGOs that can spend effectively, rather than distributing and disbursing funds to HIV/AIDS implementing agencies in all districts based in relative demand for public HIV/AIDS services". This is probably due to lack of experienced NGOs, but programs to build NGO capacity should accompany it. In Uganda, this has been seen with the PEPFAR funds where only experienced NGOs with capacity to scale up were considered for these funds. There are various ways to administer or manage an NGO (Barnet et. al, 2001) but channeling contracts through a single administrative unit in which NGOs can feel more comfortable and one that they find trustworthy is likely to be best approach. Such coordination will help to avoid the establishment of duplicate interventions by NGOs, government providers, and international agencies.

2. Accountability

Hashmat (2004) reveals that multiple donor funding demands accountability which lies at the core of NGOs' function because of the nature of their relationships with diverse stakeholders. The government provides legal cover while donors provide finance to NGOs to work with communities. Hence, NGOs are faced with diverse requirements of accountability in trends of reporting financial situation and progress to each stakeholder, thereby making accountability mechanism more complex. A number of significant policies remain among international financing entities that will require more coordinated resolution from policy makers and financial professionals if the future finance trucking is to be of quality require to assist in guiding the response to the epidemic. They include limitations on the ability of many financing entities to disaggregate projections of the future spending, either sub-sectorally or geographically. This is constrained assistance programming, where a proposal quality compares strongly with sectoral or geographic determinant in programming, financial planning is necessarily weakened.

3. Financial monitoring

Barnett et.al (2001) indicated that donor and international agencies' fiduciary responsibility to account for funds can result in administrative procedures for contracted NGOs. For example multiple bids for any purchases over a certain amount, documented salary history to justify fees charged by consultants requiring NGO staff to cosign receipts, and written receipts for all expenditure even where it is not possible.

4. Conditional grants

According to Whelan (2001), the district of Kwazul Natal in South Africa received conditional grant but experienced the following difficulties: the funds could only be used to fund the direct running costs of the programs and not the personnel and administrative costs incurred by the provincial departments. In the first year 2001, conditional grant allocations were made known to the grantee in the second half of the year. In the second year, grant allocations were made known just prior to the first half of that year. These led to delay detailed planning for HIV/AIDS health activities on the basis of complete resource envelope leading to coordination problems and in planning. Detailed planning was also rushed in the limited time before the year. In both cases, no medium term allocations were made available for the subsequent two years. The financial control structure was so difficult, such that it was difficult to truck the spending on the conditional grant component. This was so because the conditional grant components had not been allocated a separated objective code.

5. Audit requirements

Multi-donor funded programs find it costly to hire auditors to express an opinion on different sets of fund accountability statements. For example, TASO Uganda must have a minimum of 4 audited statements. USAID, EU, CDC and general purpose accounts for the general assembly. This arrangement takes a lot of time in terms of preparation, attending to the auditors and has increased costs. TASO has tried to minimize on the time taken by appointing one audit firm to carry out external audit of all the fund accountability statements, but some donor agencies like EU prefer to hire their own auditors as a condition for funding (TASO, 2001). According to TASO (1994) Memorandum and articles of association, articles 8sec7, BOT members are only empowered to recommend auditors to the general assembly for appointment.

Study methodology
In order to draw lessons from the study on the effect of donor conditions on HIV/AIDS funds towards program implementation, the methodology involves use of survey of literature to determine key donor conditions, from these conditions, an inquiry is made about level of compliance to these conditions, and how this affects program implementation. A mixed paradigm approach, with both qualitative and quantitative research techniques with cross sectional data set is purposefully obtained from both donor and implementing agencies. Respondents are agency managers-country representatives, project managers, financial managers, M&E officers, and procurement officers.

Findings
The study finds a number of donor requirements whose level of compliance is summarized in table 3.1. The problem is not with high or very high compliance but lack of compliance. Thus, table 3.1 is further reduced to investigate average weighted level of non compliance. The percentage scores on non compliance are summed for the 9 indicators and the average is got for the weighted index on compliance. From the last row, and last two columns of table 3.1, the average total of those who find 9 donor conditions not being followed are 29.9% (22.2+7.7). This percentage non compliance has a number of implications for the recipient projects. Donors may delay project funds, impose more other conditions like the need for foreign expatriates at a high cost to manage HIV/AIDS projects, and at worst the fund flow may be halted altogether.

Table 3.1 Level of compliance with standard operating procedures

Condition	Percentage response on level of compliance			
	Very high	High	Low	Very low
Finance and accounting	40	40	18	02
M&E indicators	31	28	27	24
Procurement procedures	24	29	39	08
Separate audits	66	15	18	01
Separate program reports	55	32	10	03
Separate fund accountability reports	43	30	16	11
Specific application requirement	44	45	12	03
Specific procedure of awarding grants	56	18	20	06
Specific procedure of closing a	15	33	40	12

program				
N=91			200/9=22.2	70/9=7.7

Source: *Field data collected by the researcher*

Lessons for recipient countries

1. HR-Training-Developing and maintaining a technically competent staff

-HIV/AIDS programs are dependent on the high quality staff (Oster, 1999). The work is people-intensive, thus reliance on human capital. Therefore, human capital needs must be nurtured and developed on a formal basis because of the strategies to deal with the challenge (Smillie et. al, 2007). Some NGOs lack human resource capacity to carryout M&E. Donor requirements for good quality data mean that donors continue to set up parallel system for data collection and reporting. Donors should acknowledge that not all information can or should be monitored. A few key elements should be monitored to create a constrained data set that is both manageable and informative for all stakeholders. Hulme et.al (1997) noted that…the professional skills of most NGO staff is wanting…, have weak accountability to the donors and to the grassroots. The executive Director UNAIDS, Dr. Peter Piot observes that in HIV/AIDS programs in poor countries, program managers are often little more than data processor… spending obscene amounts of time trying to satisfy dozens of duplicative reporting requirements (UNAIDS, 2004).

2. Coordination-aligning program activities with anticipated donor conditions

This includes among others, the need for strategic planning by integrating HIV/AIDS activities with other health services. Whelan (2000) shows that in the past, the HIV/AIDS prevention programs were run somewhat independently of routine public health delivery bodies. These new interventions are more complex, more dependent on participation of existing delivery structures and more resource intensive. TASO (1999) observed that a strategic plan is central to the process of working effectively for an organization. NGOs have to make strategic choices about a range of strategic priorities like deciding on which aspects of HIV/AIDS prevention, care and social, support activities to address. But in some cases, pre-existing parameters determined by donor requirements must be followed. Such parameters may include fixed allocation of funds to certain program components and areas of operation.

3. Securing special funding for staff: since most donors don't fund staff salaries but the activities the staff does.

Through for example, co-sponsoring HIV/AIDS programs to address challenges of staff funding. Some donors do not target staff salaries: Funding for staffing is problematic for many organizations. Lack of ability to pay salaries or stipends means that many organizations providing services directly in the community rely almost entirely upon volunteers. This has implications in terms of human resources turnover (volunteers who are able to find paid work is likely to take the opportunity) and a failure to build longer-term capacity and skills within an organization. A number of respondents noted that organizations that have experienced success in attracting funds come under pressure to sustain the same level of funding so as not to cut back on programs or staff. Organizations easily grow with funding, but they can't as readily shrink back to size over lean periods. There are considerable risks attached to employment of staff on a salaried basis. The challenge of meeting ever-increasing funding needs to sustain growing organizations consumes management time. With management preoccupied with organizational survival, the emphasis shifts away from developing programs and delivering services. 'Now it's no longer about servicing the community and HIV affecting and infecting the people, it's about us, it's about the institution. It's no longer about the people outside there - no, it's about us inside the institution.' When staff needs to be laid off, resulting conflicts about who retains jobs may result in severe distraction from the primary organizational objectives. At least in one case, this has led to chronic and unresolved interpersonal conflicts which consume an inordinate amount of time. In South Africa's HIV'AIDS community audit, most organizations touched upon one or more of the following issues:(1) the general shortage of staff and volunteers, which leads to stress and heavy workloads; (2) the need for more training and capacity building of staff and volunteers; and (3) the need for more financial support and/or incentives for both volunteers and staff, but particularly volunteers. Problems with remuneration of staff and volunteers are acute and multi-faceted. Many organizations noted the need to give volunteers incentives: many of them are poor, some are prone to becoming sick, and in many cases are also required to arrange their own transport (Nandin, 2007).

4. Need to have an agreement between the donor and recipient country

Where different donors for the same cause, fund an implementing agency, the donors and the grantee should agree to the same set of minimum guidelines through a combined "memorandum of understanding" on the requirements expected from the grantee and also on the requirements to be fulfilled by each donor. This would call for 'pooled funding with specific reporting requirements' including fund accountability statements and financial statements whereby all donors use the same reports and share the same program output/results.

5. Continuous evaluation of internal capacity

An implementing agency should continuously evaluate its internal capacity to deliver the planned services. This helps the grantee to gauge whether more grants/funds for additional activities from a different donor can be absorbed at the right pace. Without the right internal capacity, the relationship, conditions and requirements become more complicated.

References

1. Adam, C. and J. W. Gunning (2002). "*Redesigning the Aid Contract*: Donors' Use of Performance Indicators in Uganda." World Development 30(12): 2045 - 2056.
2. Barnet et al, (2001) contracting for Non Governmental organization to combat HIV. Special Initiative Report No.33
3. Bennett S, et al, (2006); Scaling up HIV/AIDS Evaluation. Lancet 367 (9504): 79-82.
4. Broback U and Sjolander S (2002); Program support and public financial management: a new role for bilateral donors in poverty strategy work. Stockholm: SIDA studies number 6, 2007.
5. Brugha R, et al. (2004): The Global Fund: managing great expectations. Lancet 364: 95-100.
6. CDC (2002): Facts for public health personnel; male latex condoms and sexually transmitted diseases, http://www.cdc.gov/hiv/mmr/pubs/facts/condoms.htm.
7. Guthrie, G. & Hickey, A. (2004). *Funding the fight: Budgeting for HIV and AIDS in developing countries.* Cape Town, IDASA AIDS Budget Unit. www.idasa.org.za.
8. MacAdam, M. 2003. Uganda Offers Hope: Beating AIDS in Africa. www.sustainabletimes.ca/articles/aidsinafrica.htm, accessed on 2 March 2003.
9. Oomman N (2005): An overview of the World Bank's Response to the HIV/AIDS Epidemic in Africa, with a focus on the Multi-Country HIV./AIDS Program (MAP), Centre for Global Development, World Bank.
10. Oomman, N., et al. (2007). Following the Funding for HIV/AIDS: A Comparative Analysis of the Funding Practices of PEPFAR, the Global Fund and World Bank MAP in Mozambique, Uganda and Zambia. Washington, Center for Global Development.
11. Siamwiza R (2007): Analysis of Financing for the National HIV and AIDS Response: Civil Society Component.
12. TASO (2003): Strategic Plan 2003-2007
13. The Global Fund (2006) "The Global Fund Welcomes Ugandan Corruption Inquiry Report." The Global Fund Press Release - 2 June 2006 Volume, DOI:
14. UNAIDS & WHO (1998): Global HIV/AIDS epidemic, Geneva
15. UNAIDS (2003): Report on the state of HIV/AIDS financing
16. UNAIDS (2004): Report on the global AIDS epidemic
17. UNAIDS (2004a). *Funding for AIDS – Factsheet.* Geneva, UNAIDS.
18. UNAIDS (2004b); The 'Three Ones': Driving concerted action on AIDS at country level. Geneva, UNAIDS. www.unaids.org.

19. UNAIDS (2005a) Intensifying HIV Prevention: UNAIDS Policy Position Paper, Geneva.
20. UNAIDS (2005b) AIDS Epidemic Update: Special Report on HIV, Geneva.
21. UNAIDS. (2004c). Report on the global AIDS epidemic. Geneva, UNAIDS.
22. UNAIDS/OECD (2004): Analysis of aid in support of HIV/AIDS control. Geneva, UNAIDS.
23. UNAIDS/WHO (2006) AIDS Epidemic Update.
24. UNICEF (1992): New phase of UNICEF support for AIDS control in Uganda. Project document, Kampala
25. Whelan P. & A. Hickey (2001): "sources and methods of funding the health sector response to HIV/AIDS. Report by Idasa" budget information service.
26. Whelan P. (2001): HIV/AIDS Financing; institute of democracy in South Africa http://.www.hst.org.za/sahr/2001/chapt8htm
27. World Bank (2006) Health financing revisited a practitioner's guide. Paris declaration and aid effectiveness; High level forum (2005) ownership, harmonization, alignment, results and mutual accountability; Joint progress towards enhanced aid effectiveness.
28. World Health Organization (2005) The World health Report 2005: Making every child and mother count.

YOUR KNOWLEDGE HAS VALUE

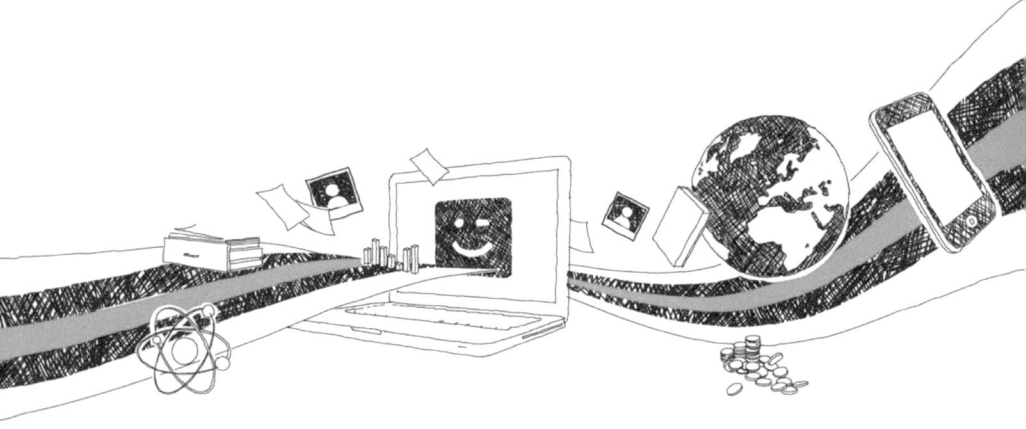

- We will publish your bachelor's and master's thesis, essays and papers

- Your own eBook and book - sold worldwide in all relevant shops

- Earn money with each sale

Upload your text at www.GRIN.com
and publish for free

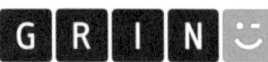